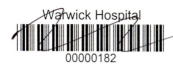

# Self-assessment picture tests
# Medicine
## Volume 3

## Pierre-Marc Bouloux
BSc MD FRCP

**Reader in Endocrinology**
**Department of Endocrinology**
Royal Free Hospital
London

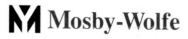 Mosby-Wolfe

London • Baltimore • Barcelona • Bogotá • Boston
Buenos Aires • Carlsbad, CA • Chicago • Madrid
Mexico City • Milan • Naples, FL • New York
Philadelphia • St. Louis • Seoul • Singapore
Sydney • Taipei • Tokyo • Toronto • Wiesbaden

| | |
|---|---|
| Publisher: | **Richard Furn** |
| Development Editor: | **Jennifer Prast** |
| Project Manager: | **Linda Horrell, Jane Tozer** |
| Production: | **Gudrun Hughes** |
| Index: | **Angela Cottingham** |
| Layout: | **Lindy van den Berghe** |
| Cover Design: | **Greg Smith** |

# Preface

Much of clinical practice consists of pattern recognition, and the ability to detect swiftly and interpret physical signs correctly is at the heart of the diagnostic process (and indeed a prequisite for passing clinical examinations!). In these four volumes, I have compiled 800 examples of common and not so common clinical problems covering wide areas of medicine. The format is simple, unambiguous and unpretentious: a photographic plate with a short question, or questions, relating to the physical sign or underlying diagnosis. The aim is to challenge the reader's diagnostic skills. I have annotated the answer in many cases to give the reader some background information about the condition illustrated. These volumes should be seen as an adjunct to existing illustrated textbooks of clinical medicine such as Forbes/Jackson *Color Atlas and Text of Clinical Medicine,* 2nd edition.

# Acknowledgements

I would like to acknowledge the wonderful assistance given to me by the Department of Medical Illustrations at the Royal Free Hospital School of Medicine, and the excellent support of Miss Patsy Coskeran in assembling the material.

To Jane, Dominic, Matthew, Natalie and my late brother Alain

**1 ▶**

This lady presented with a long history of generalized pruritus and a persistently raised alkaline phosphatase. There had been a change in her skin colour. What is the likely diagnosis?

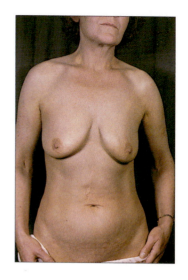

**2 ▶**

(a) What is the diagnosis?
(b) List two causes of pain in the hand in this condition.

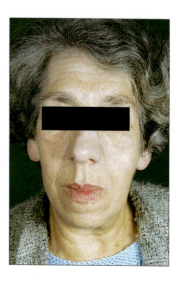

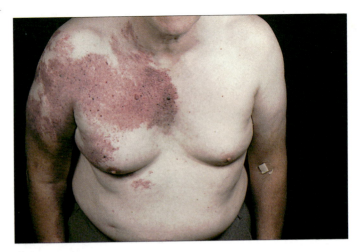

▲ 3
What two physical signs are shown in this slide?

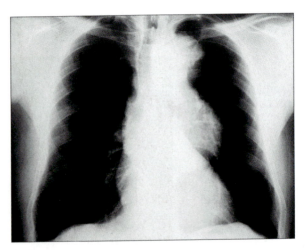

▲ 4
This is the chest radiograph of a patient who complained
of a sudden onset of chest pain radiating to the back.
What is the diagnosis?

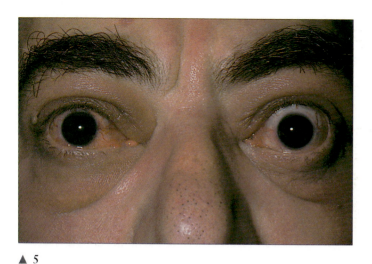

▲ 5
(a) What is the diagnosis?
(b) What surgical intervention has previously been carried out in
   this patient?

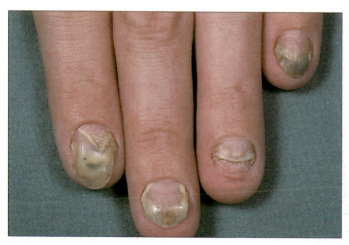

▲ 6
List three possible causes of this appearance.

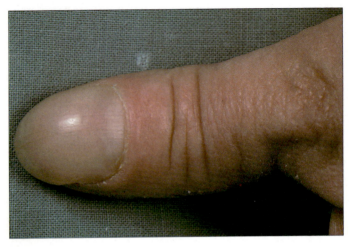

▲ 7
This patient commented that her fingers had assumed an abnormal curvature over a period of two years. There were some nodular itchy lesions in her pretibial regions. What is the diagnosis?

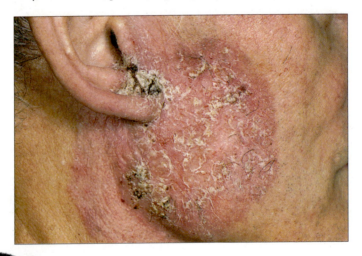

8
...sion was getting slowly larger in size and had been present ... What is the diagnosis?

**9** ▶

These are the legs of a patient who also complained of tenderness in his arms and legs, and easy gum bleeding. What diagnosis is suggested?

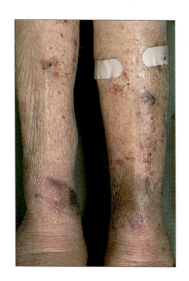

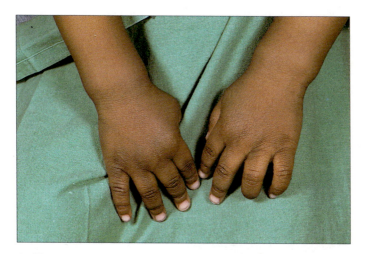

▲ **10**

These are the hands of a little girl with short stature and generalized weakness and hypotonia. Her wrists were particularly sore. What diagnosis is suggested?

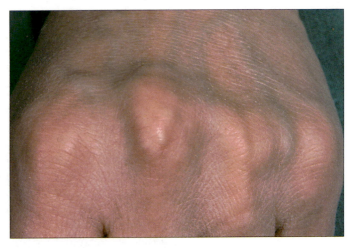

▲ 11

(a) What physical sign is shown?

(b) What investigations should be performed?

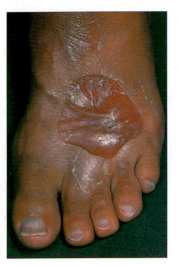

◀ 12

This patient easily developed bullo vesicular lesions on exposure to sunlight. What diagnosis is suggested?

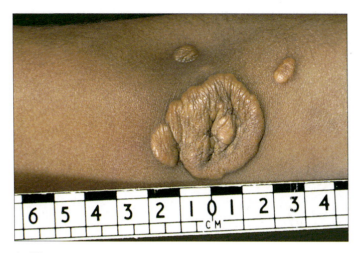

▲ 13
What lesion is shown?

14 ▶
What abnormality is shown on
this man's legs?

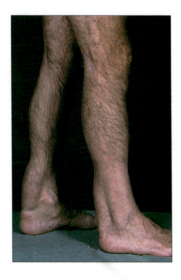

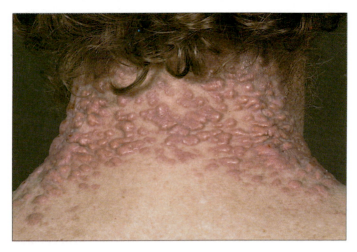

▲ 15

What is the diagnosis?

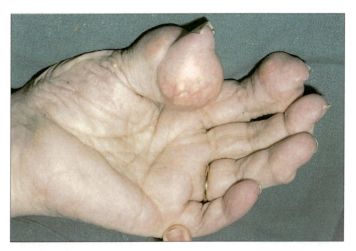

▲ 16

(a) What is the diagnosis?

(b) What biochemical abnormality should be sought?

**17 ▶**
List two
abnormalities.

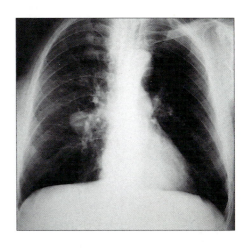

**18 ▶**
What abnormality
is shown on this
radiograph?

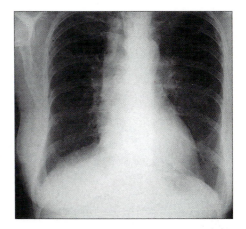

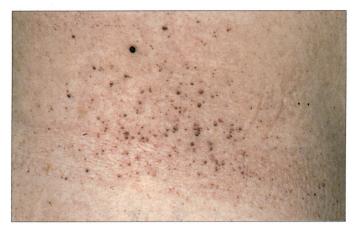

▲ 19
This patient had renal disease. What diagnosis is suggested by this appearance?

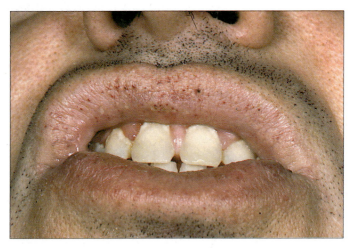

▲ 20
Several lesions were present both on this man's lip and on his scrotum. He had additional lesions on his buttocks. What is the diagnosis?

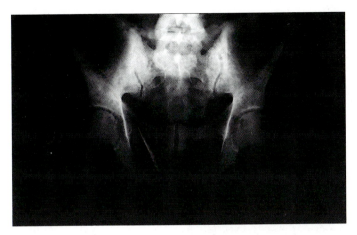

▲ 21
This man had carcinoma of the prostate. What lesions are shown?

22 ▶
What abnormality
is shown on this
right lateral
radiograph?

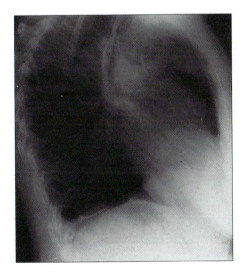

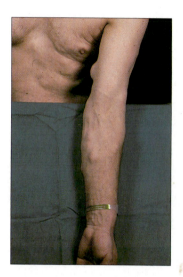

**◄ 23**
These lesions had been present over a long period of time. Suggest two possible diagnoses.

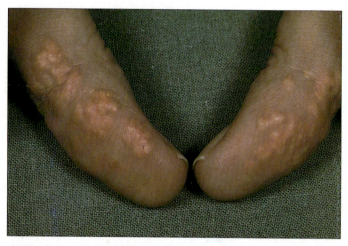

**▲ 24**
What causes this appearance?

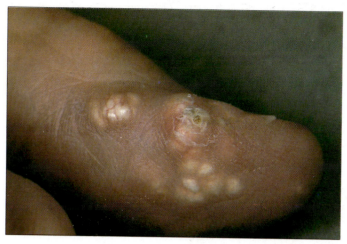

**▲ 25**

This patient had renal insufficiency. What is the likely cause of this appearance?

**26 ▶**

These are the legs of a man who has a glomerulonephritic illness and arthralgia. He also had hepatosplenomegaly. What is the most likely diagnosis?

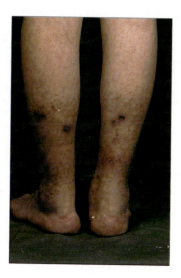

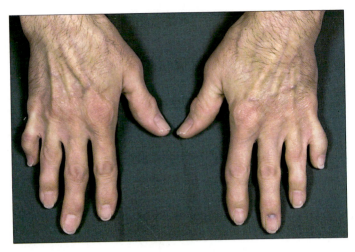

▲ 27
This man was under investigation for abnormal extrapyramidal movements and tetany. What diagnosis is suggested?

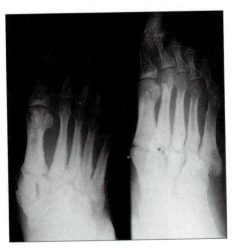

◀ 28
The deformities shown were totally painless. What diagnosis is suggested?

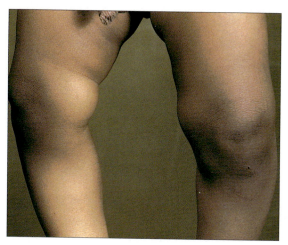

▲ 29
What abnormality is shown?

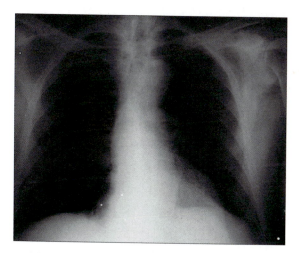

▲ 30
This man was under investigation for a persistently raised alkaline phosphatase. What is the diagnosis?

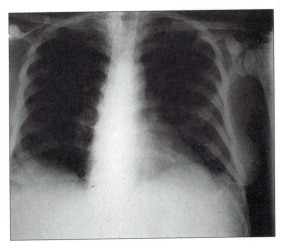

▲ 31
This man was receiving a depot gonadotrophin releasing hormone (GnRH) preparation for a chronic disease. What is the likely underlying cause?

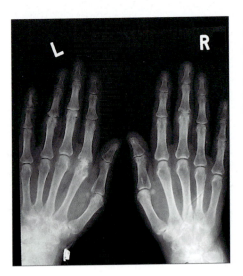

◀ 32
What is the most likely cause of the appearances shown on these radiographs of the hands?

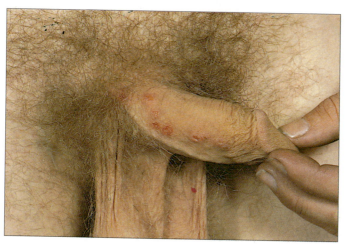

▲ 33

(a) What lesion is shown?
(b) How may it be treated?

34 ▶

What lesion is shown?

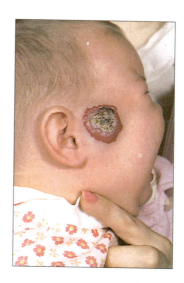

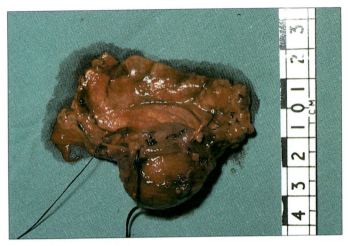

▲ 35
This lesion was removed from the adrenal of a hypertensive patient. What is the most likely diagnosis?

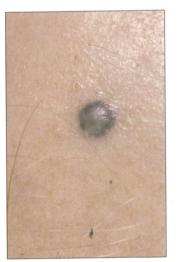

◄ 36
What lesion is shown on this scalp?

**37** ▶

This lesion had been present since birth. What is it?

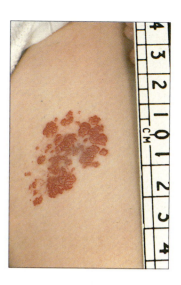

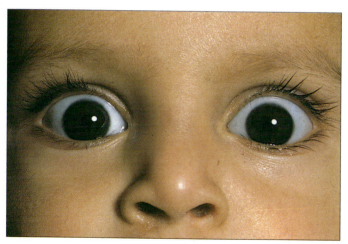

▲ **38**

This child had diarrhoea. What is the diagnosis?

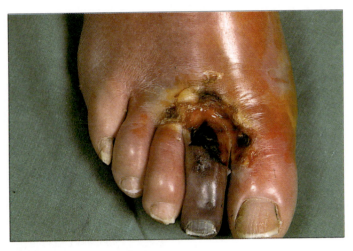

▲ 39

This is the foot of a diabetic man following a fairly trivial injury. What should be excluded?

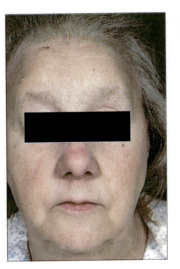

◄ 40

(a) What diagnosis is suggested by this appearance?

(b) List three neurological complications of this condition.

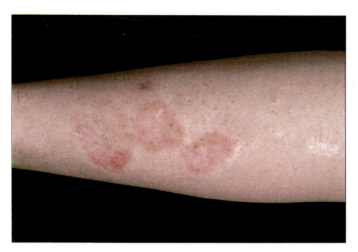

▲ 41
What lesion is shown on the shin of this diabetic patient?

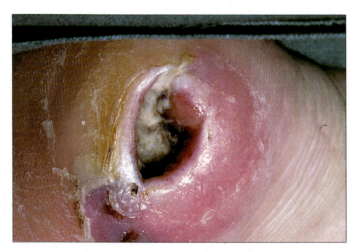

▲ 42
What diagnosis is suggested by this appearance?

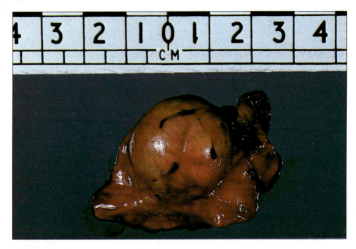

▲ 43
This is an adrenal resection specimen from a patient with hypokalaemia and alkalosis. What would you expect the plasma renin activity to be?

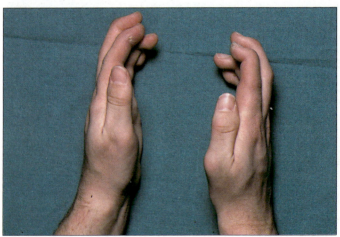

▲ 44
These are the hands of a diabetic. What physical sign is shown?

**45** ▶
These are oval pigmented
lesions appearing on the legs of
a diabetic patient being treated
with insulin. What is the name
of these lesions?

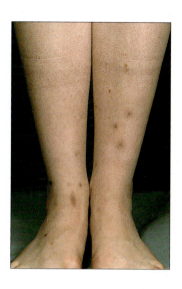

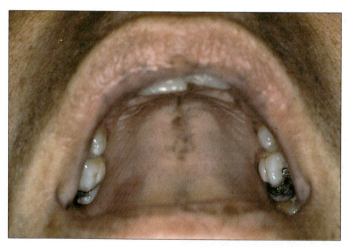

▲ **46**
This is the mouth of a man who had lost weight and was
complaining of persistent nausea. His liver function tests were
abnormal. What diagnosis should be excluded?

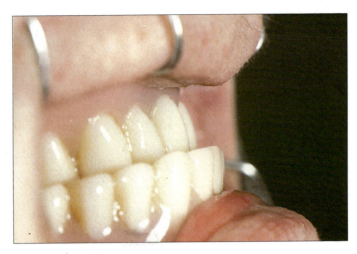

▲ 47
What is the diagnosis?

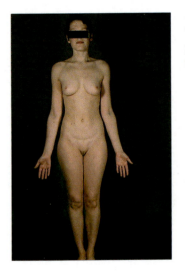

◄ 48
This patient presented with primary amenorrhoea. What is the diagnosis?

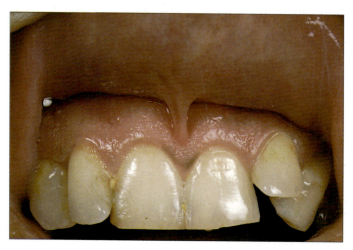

▲ 49
The biochemistry of this man showed hypokalaemia, hyponatraemia, and raised urea. What is the likely diagnosis?

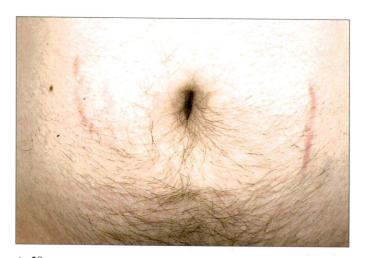

▲ 50
(a) What physical sign is shown?
(b) List two associations.

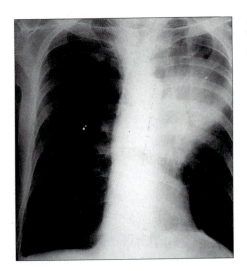

◀ 51
What is the
diagnosis?

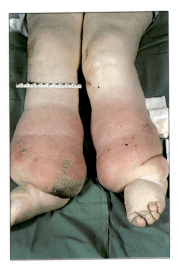

◀ 52
What is the diagnosis?

**53 ▶**
This patient was being investigated for copious sputum production and clubbing. What is the most likely diagnosis?

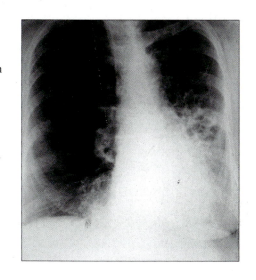

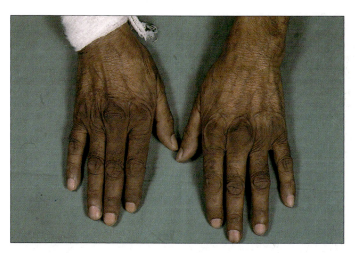

**▲ 54**
This pigmentation was present in sun exposed areas. What is the most likely diagnosis?

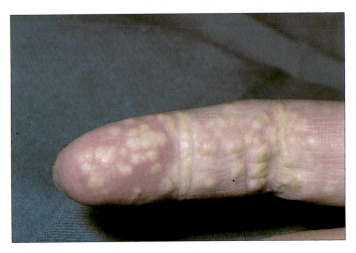

▲ 55
What is the most likely cause of this appearance?

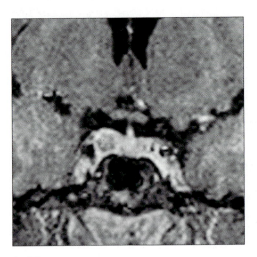

▲ 56
What is the diagnosis?

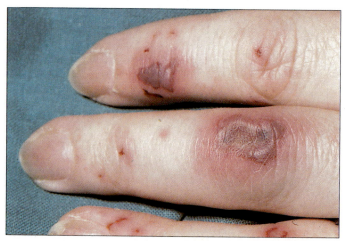

▲ 57
This is the hand of a patient in an intensive care unit who was being treated for a life-threatening condition. What is the likely diagnosis?

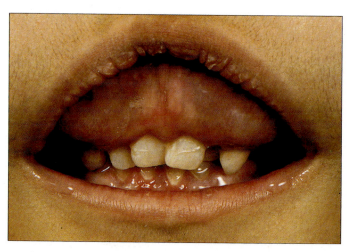

▲ 58
This is the mouth of a child receiving regular blood transfusions for an anaemia. What is the most likely diagnosis?

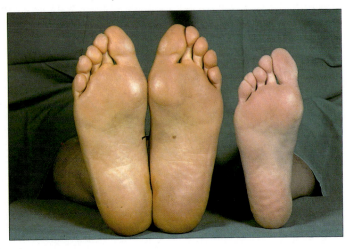

▲ 59

These are the feet of a patient who took large quantities of substances from a health food store. A normal foot is shown for comparison. What is the most likely diagnosis?

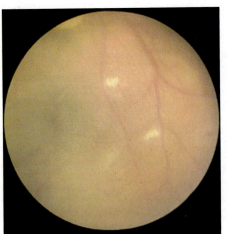

◀ 60

This man with known acquired immune deficiency syndrome (AIDS) complained of reduced visual acuity. What diagnosis should be suspected from this appearance?

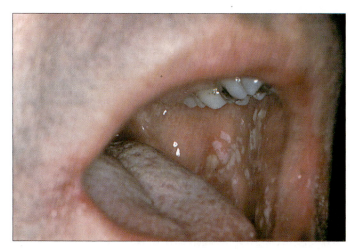

▲ 61

What is the most likely cause of this appearance?

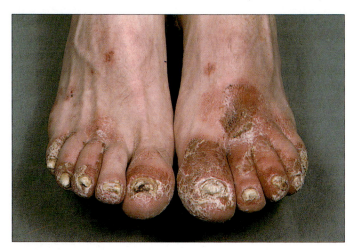

▲ 62

What is the cause of this appearance?

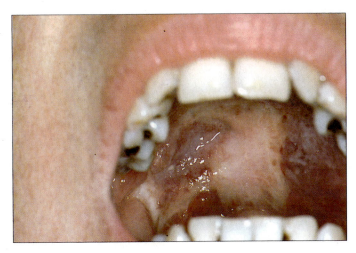

▲ 63
This is the oral appearance of a man with AIDS. What is the most likely diagnosis?

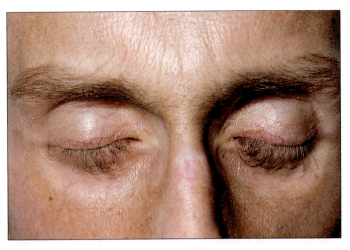

▲ 64
(a) What physical sign is shown?
(b) Cite one association.

## 65 ▶

List two potential causes of this appearance.

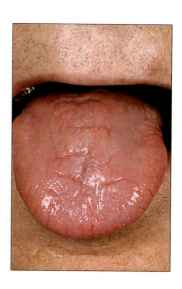

## 66 ▶

List two possible causes of this facial appearance.

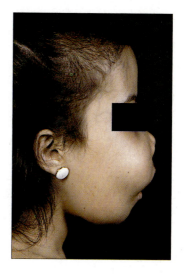

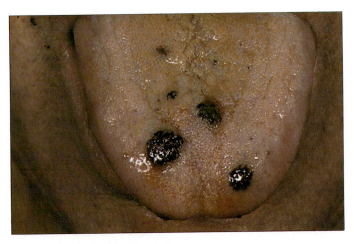

▲ 67
With what haematological abnormality are these physical signs likely to be associated?

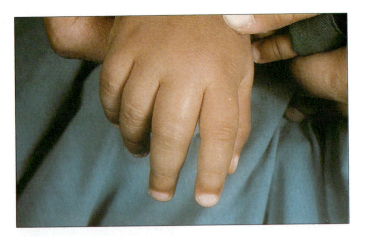

▲ 68
This is the hand of a patient with an anaemia and recurrent tenderness of the fingers.
(a) What physical sign is shown?
(b) What is the likely underlying diagnosis?

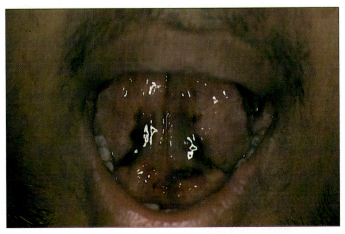

▲ 69
This is the appearance of the mouth of a man who had had multiple haemarthroses and contraction deformities. What is the most likely diagnosis?

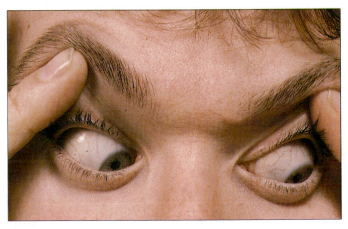

▲ 70
This patient is attempting to look downwards and to the left. Diplopia was present. What the most likely diagnosis?

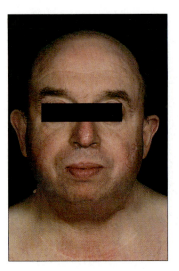

**◄ 71**
This man was known to have chronic hypocalcaemia and also had brachydactyly. What does his appearance suggest?

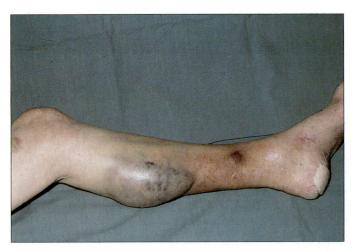

**▲ 72**
What is the diagnosis?

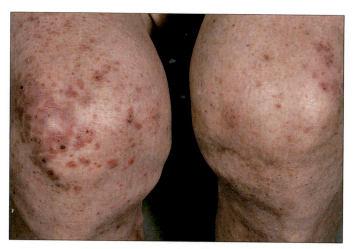

▲ 73

This eruption appeared some eight days after the taking a sulphonamide. What is the most likely diagnosis?

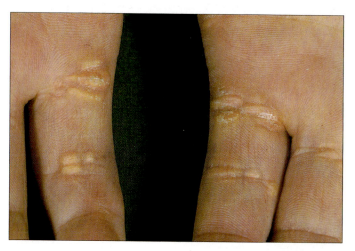

▲ 74

What physical sign is shown?

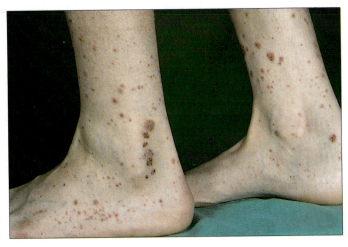

▲ 75

In addition to this cutaneous rash, this patient complained of lower abdominal pain. What is the most likely diagnosis?

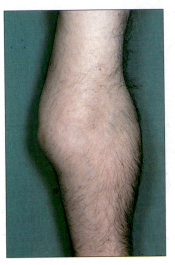

◀ 76
This was a painless deformity. What is the most likely diagnosis?

**77** ▶

This eruption was present in a man with diabetes, insipidus, and an anaemia. What is the likely diagnosis?

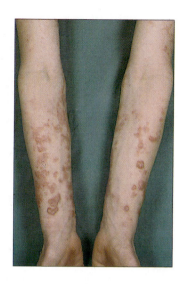

**78** ▶
What is the diagnosis?

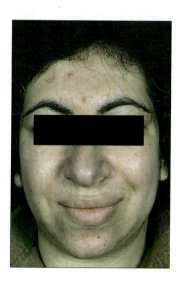

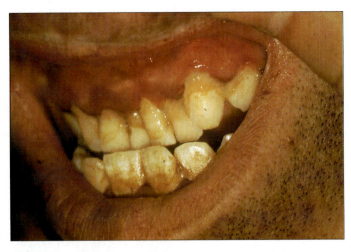

▲ 79

This man was under investigation for purpuric eruptions. What is the most likely diagnosis?

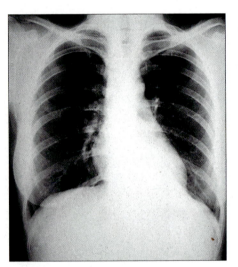

◀ 80
This is the chest radiograph of a patient with weight loss and a cough. What radiological abnormality is shown?

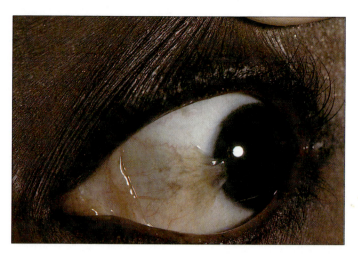

▲ 81
What physical sign is shown?

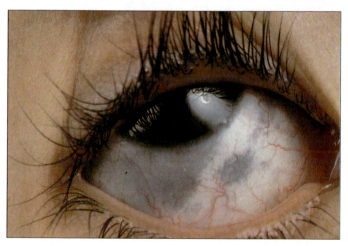

▲ 82
What physical sign is shown?

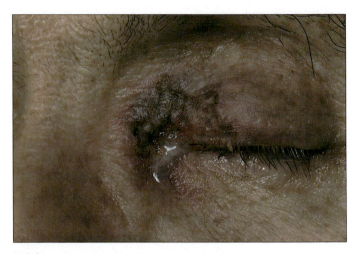

▲ 83
What is the diagnosis?

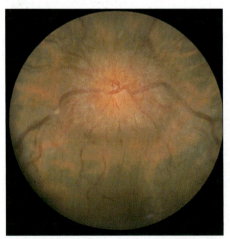

◀ 84
What is the
diagnosis?

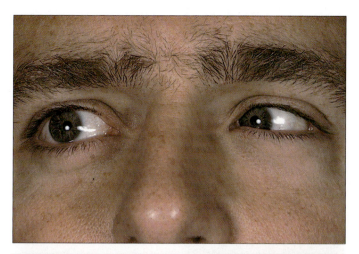

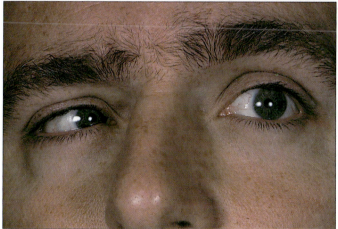

▲ 85
What is the likely diagnosis?

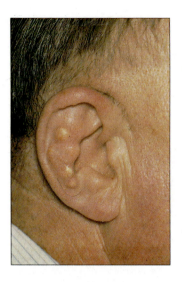

◀ 86
This patient's other ear was similarly affected, and he had pain in his nose. What is the diagnosis?

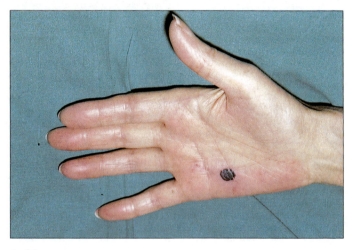

▲ 87
This lesion was exquisitely tender and the patient had a pyrexia of unknown origin. What is the most likely diagnosis?

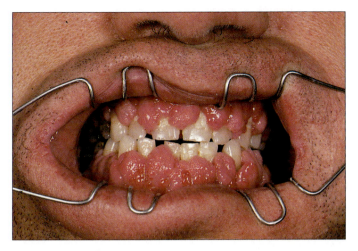

▲ 88
(a) What physical sign is shown?
(b) List two associations.

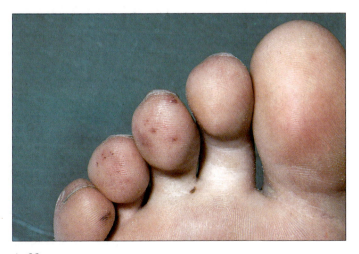

▲ 89
This patient had microscopic haematuria and weight loss. What diagnosis is suggested by these appearances?

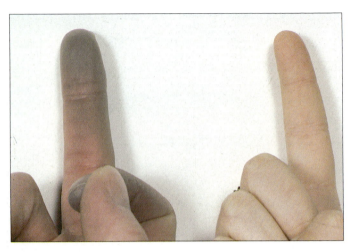

▲ 90
The hand on the right is a control hand. What physical sign is shown on the left?

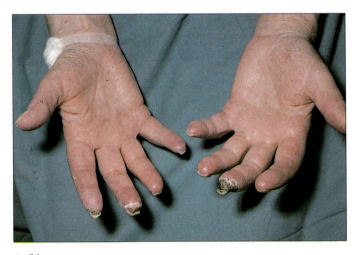

▲ 91
This patient complained of recurrent episodes of painful hands. What diagnosis is suggested by these appearances?

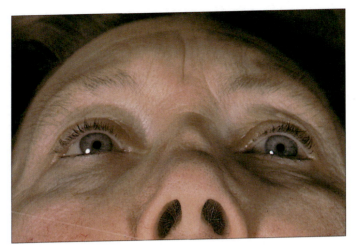

▲ 92
This patient presented with haematuria and haemoptysis. What diagnosis is suggested?

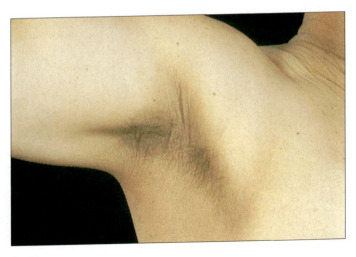

▲ 93
(a) What physical sign is shown?
(b) List two associations.

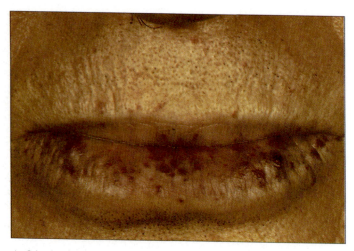

▲ 94
(a) What physical sign is shown?
(b) What internal complications occur?

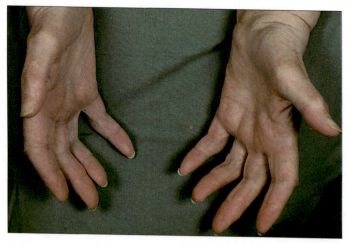

▲ 95
With what neurological lesions are these appearances associated?

What is the diagnosis?

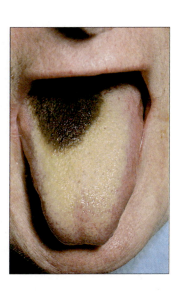

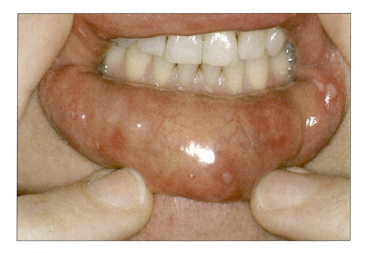

▲ 97
These lesions were very painful. The patient had abdominal pain
and occasional bouts of diarrhoea. What diagnosis is suggested?

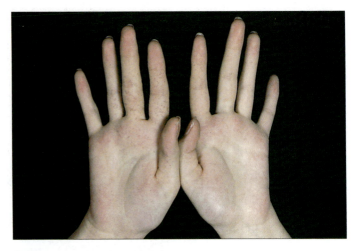

▲ 98
(a) What physical sign is shown?
(b) List three associations.

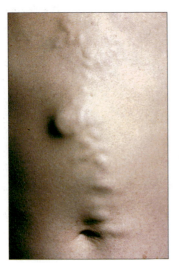

◀ 99
What is the most likely cause of this appearance?

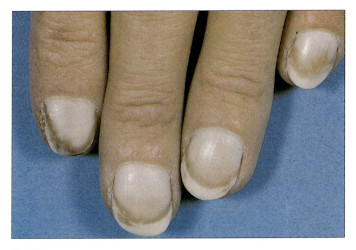

▲ 100
(a) What physical sign is shown?
(b) List two associations.

101 ▶
This patient had severe
dyslipidaemia. What is the most
likely diagnosis?

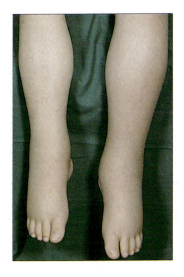

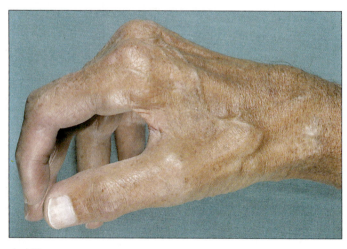

▲ 102
What two physical signs are demonstrated?

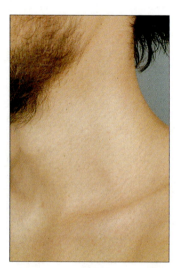

◄ 103
This man had cataracts and hypogonadism. What is the most likely diagnosis?

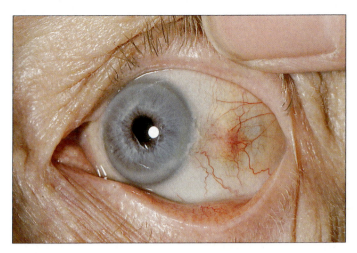

▲ 104
(a) What physical sign is shown?
(b) List two associations.

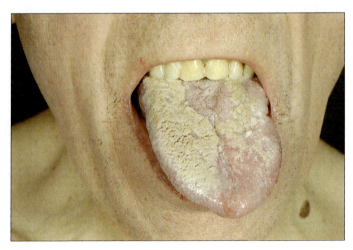

▲ 105
What physical sign is shown?

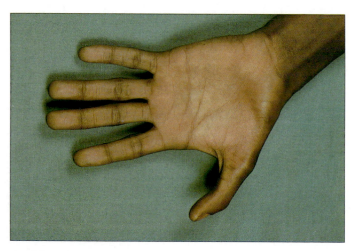

▲ 106

(a) What physical sign is shown?

(b) With what root value is this lesion associated?

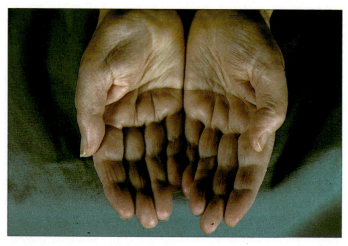

▲ 107

(a) What is the most likely cause of this appearance?

(b) List two associations.

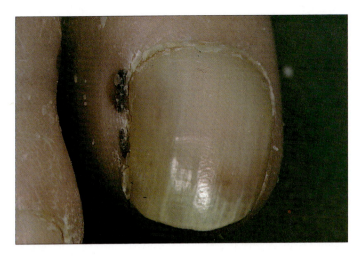

▲ 108
(a) What two physical signs are shown?
(b) What underlying diagnosis is suggested?

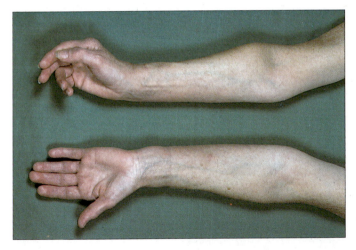

▲ 109
These are the hands of a diabetic patient. What lesion is likely to account for this appearance?

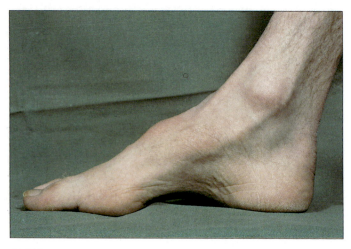

▲ 110
With what root value is this lesion likely to be associated?

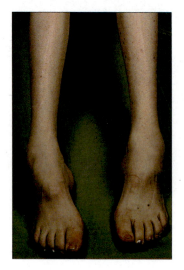

◀ 111
This lesion was present in the lower and upper limbs, and had been present for over two decades. It did not appear to be progressive. There is a family history of this condition. What is the likely diagnosis?

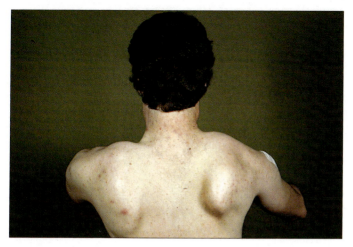

▲ 112
(a) What physical sign is shown?
(b) With what lesion is it usually associated?

113 ▶
What endocrine abnormalities
are associated with this
condition?

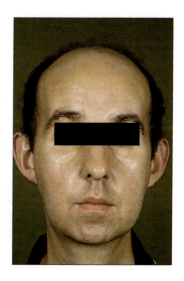

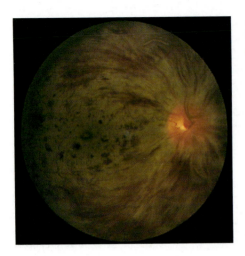

◀ 114
What is the
diagnosis?

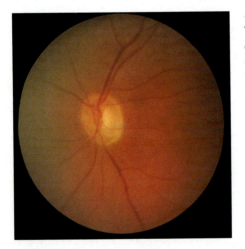

◀ 115
This patient
complained of
sudden loss of
vision. What is the
likely cause?

**116** ▶
(a) What lesion is shown?
(b) List two associations.

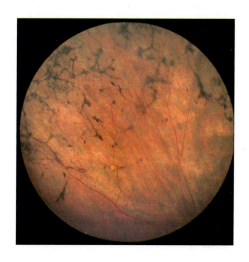

▶ **117**
This was an incidental finding on fundoscopy. The patient was totally asymptomatic. What is the diagnosis?

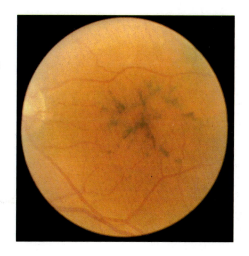

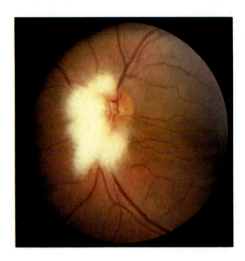

◄ 118
What lesion is
shown?

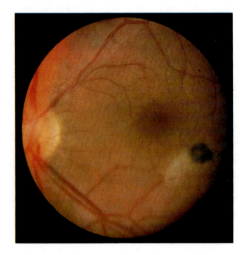

◄ 119
(a) What lesion is
shown?
(b) List two
associations.

**120 ▶**
What lesion is
shown?

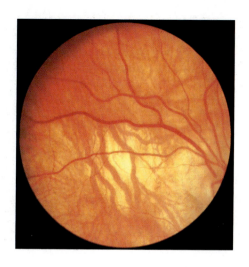

**121 ▶**
This was an
incidental
appearance. What is
the diagnosis?

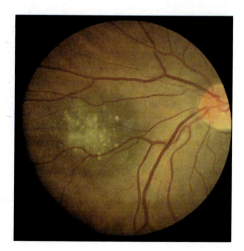

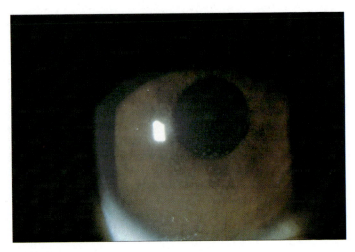

▲ 122

This patient presented with floaters. What is the diagnosis?

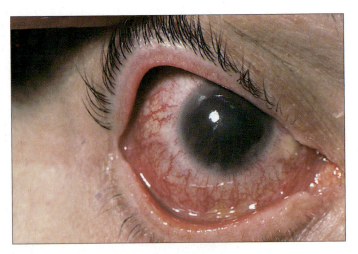

▲ 123

This patient complained of pain in the eye and seeing haloes around objects. What is the diagnosis?

**124** ▶
What is the most likely underlying diagnosis?

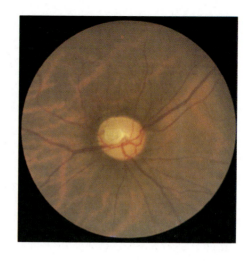

**125** ▶
This patient had a blow to the eye. What lesion is shown?

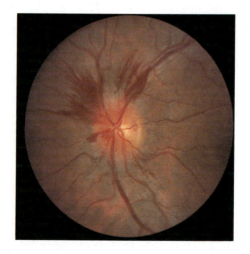

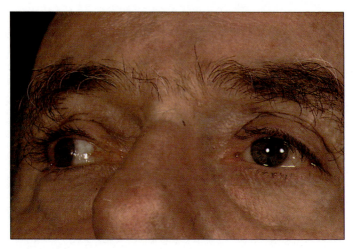

▲ 126
This patient complained of an acute onset of double vision on looking to the right. What is the cause?

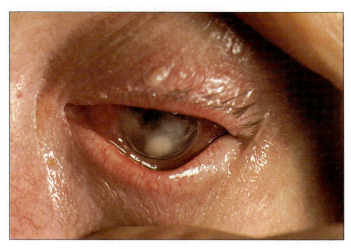

▲ 127
What is the diagnosis?

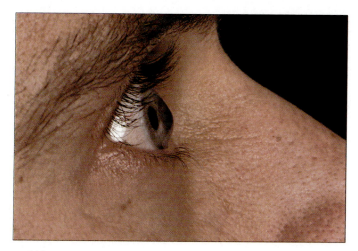

▲ **128**
(a) What is the diagnosis?
(b) Cite one association.

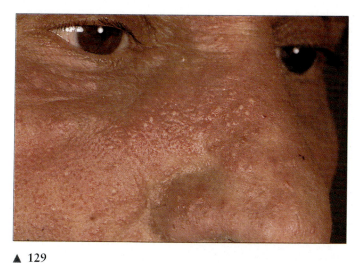

▲ **129**
(a) What lesion is shown?
(b) List three predisposing factors.

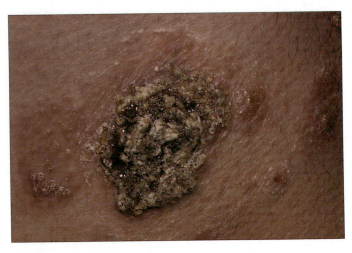

▲ 130
These lesions spread rather rapidly over the skin. What is the diagnosis?

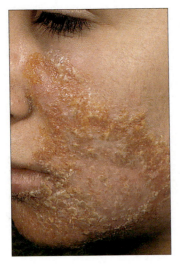

◄ 131
What is the diagnosis?

**132** ▶

This lesion had been present for a number of months. What is it?

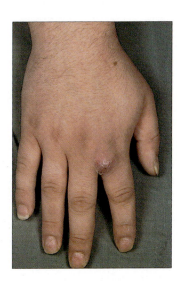

**133** ▶

(a) What lesion is shown?
(b) List two associations.

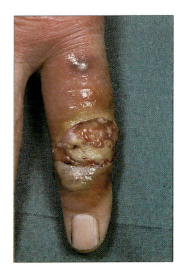

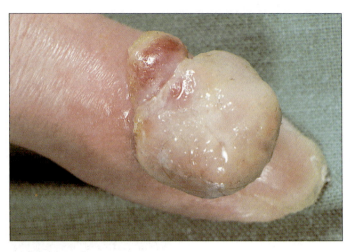

▲ 134
What is the diagnosis?

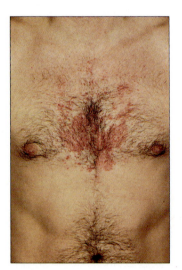

◄ 135
What is the diagnosis?

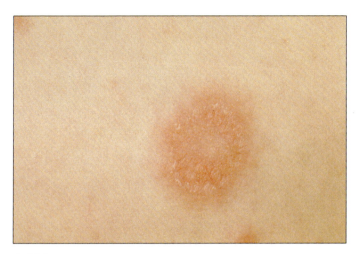

▲ 136
What is the diagnosis?

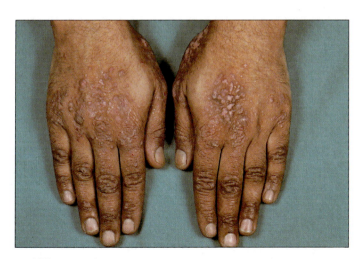

▲ 137
These nodular lesions were previously itchy. What is the likely diagnosis?

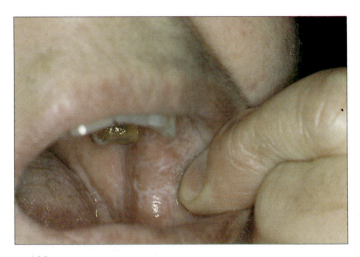

▲ 138
What is the most likely diagnosis?

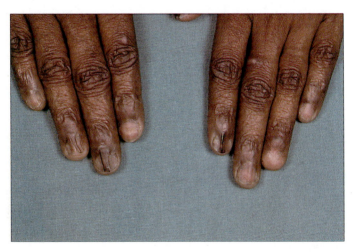

▲ 139
What is the most likely diagnosis?

**140** ▶
What is the most likely cause of
this chronic lesion?

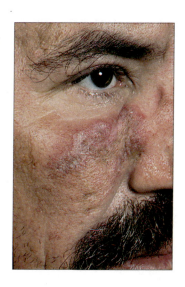

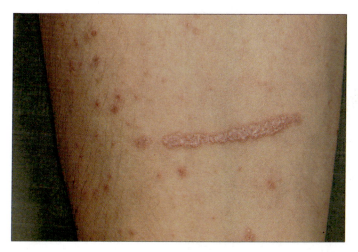

▲ **141**
What is the diagnosis?

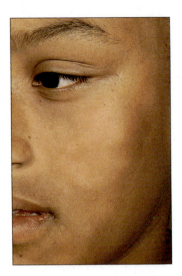

◄ 142
What is the lesion?

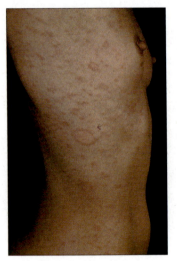

◄ 143
What is the diagnosis?

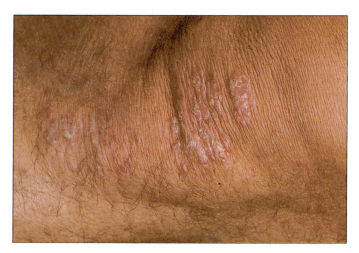

▲ 144
What is the most likely diagnosis?

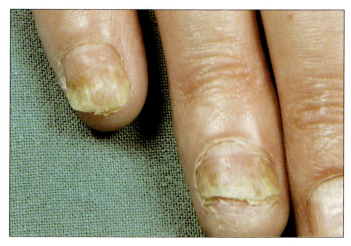

▲ 145
What is the most likely cause of these nail changes?

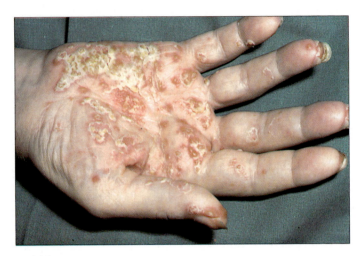

▲ 146

What is the most likely cause of this appearance?

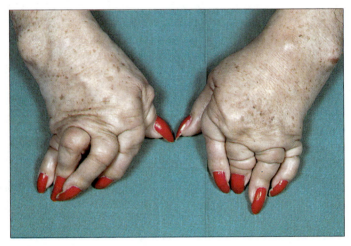

▲ 147

What is the most likely cause of this deformity?

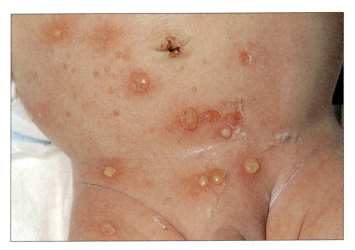

▲ 148
These lesions were present on the abdomen of a neonate. What is
the most likely diagnosis?

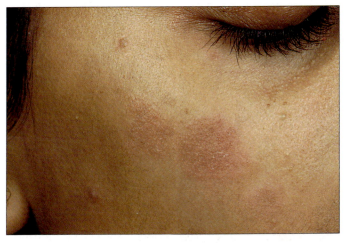

▲ 149
This patient had presented originally with some hair loss and
cicatricial lesions on her head. This lesion then appeared. What is
the most likely diagnosis?

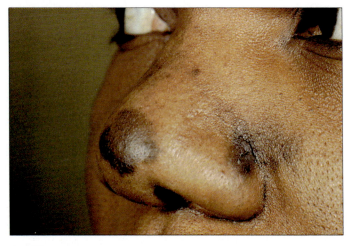

▲ 150
What is the most likely cause of these lesions?

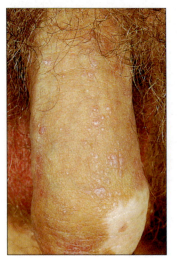

◄ 151
What is the most likely cause of
these penile lesions?

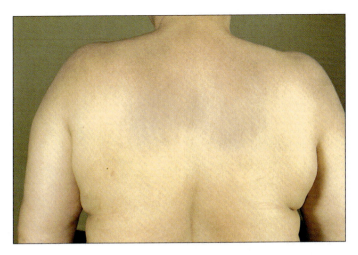

**▲ 152**
What diagnosis is suggested by these lesions?

**153 ▶**
What is the diagnosis?

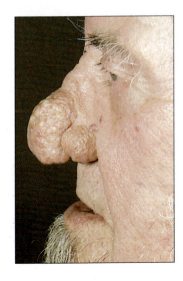

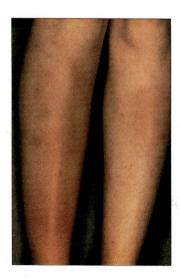

◄ 154
These lesions were tender. What is the diagnosis?

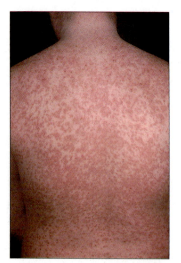

◄ 155
This patient had recently started carbamazepine therapy. What is the diagnosis?

**156** ▶
This patient had severe pyrexia with a high neutrophil count. Some oral lesions were present. What is the most likely diagnosis?

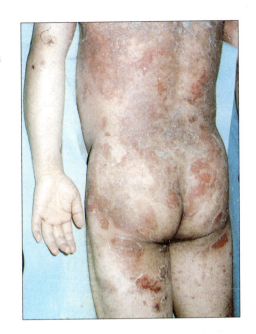

**157** ▶
What is the most likely cause of this appearance?

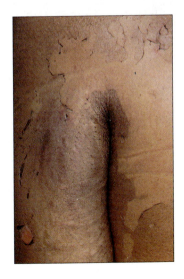

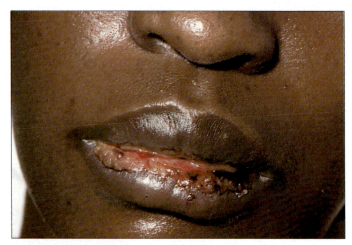

▲ 158

In addition to generalized cutaneous lesions, the mucous membranes appear to be affected in this patient. What is the most likely diagnosis?

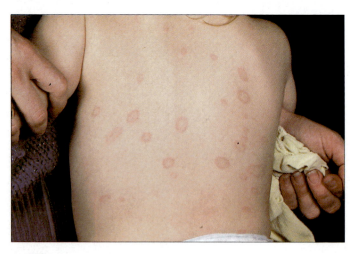

▲ 159
What lesion is shown?

160 ▶
What is the diagnosis?

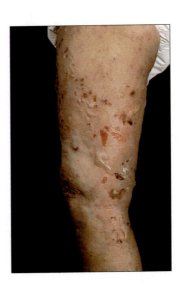

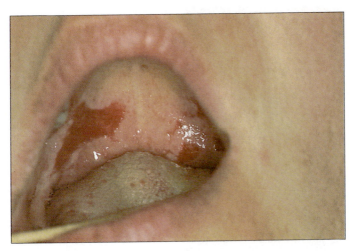

▲ 161
Superficial skin denudation was seen on this patient's body. What is the most likely diagnosis?

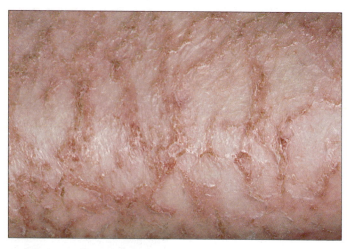

▲ 162
What is the diagnosis?

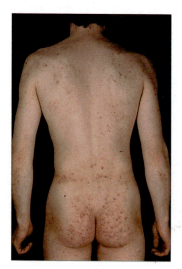

◄ 163
This was an intensely itchy eruption. What is the most likely diagnosis?

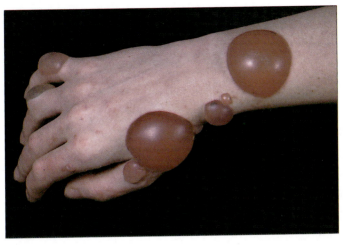

▲ 164
This patient presented with these lesions a short time after taking a trip into a forest. What is the most likely diagnosis?

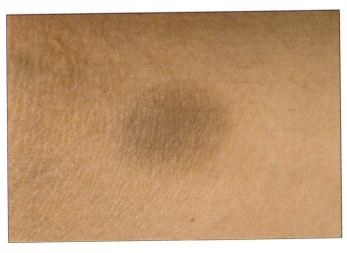

▲ 165
This patient was taking a laxative regularly. What is the most likely cause of this lesion?

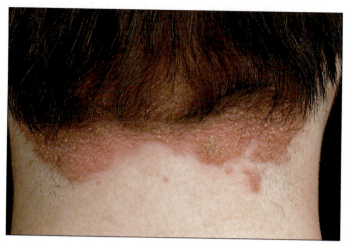

▲ 166

This patient had recently had her hair dyed. What is the most likely cause of this appearance?

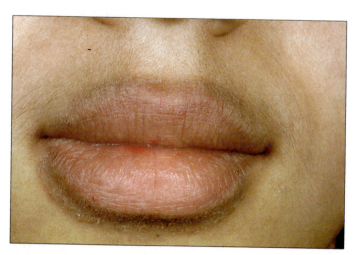

▲ 167

What is the diagnosis?

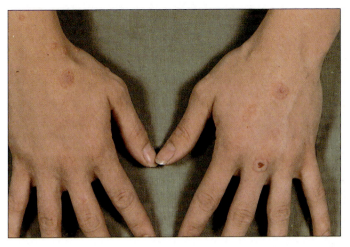

▲ 168
These lesions had occurred on a number of occasions over a period of one year. What is the most likely diagnosis?

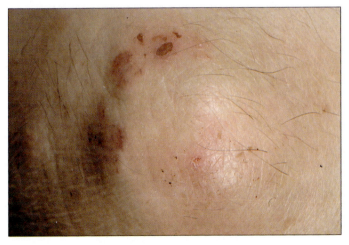

▲ 169
These are intensely itchy lesions. What is the most likely diagnosis?

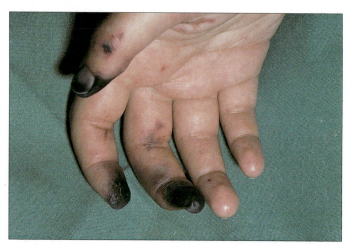

▲ 170
What is the most likely cause of this appearance?

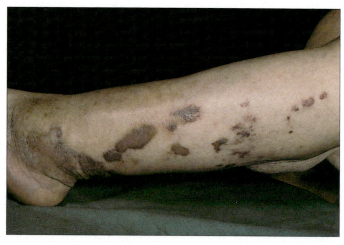

▲ 171
What is the most likely cause of this appearance?

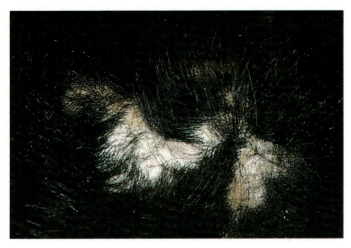

▲ 172
What is the most likely cause of this appearance?

173 ▶
What is the likely diagnosis?

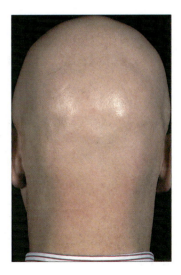

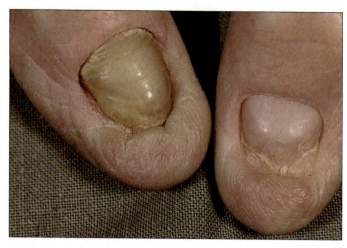

▲ 174

This patient was being investigated for a pleural effusion. What is the most likely diagnosis?

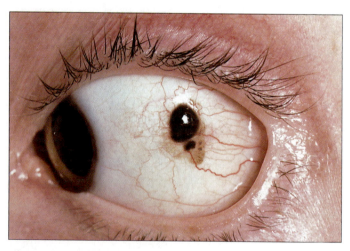

▲ 175

What is the diagnosis?

**176** ▶
What is the diagnosis?

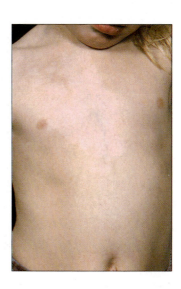

**177** ▶
What is the most likely cause of
this appearance?

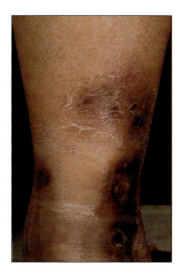

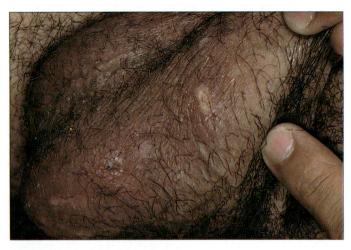

▲ 178

These were painful lesions, and others were present in the mouth. What is the most likely diagnosis?

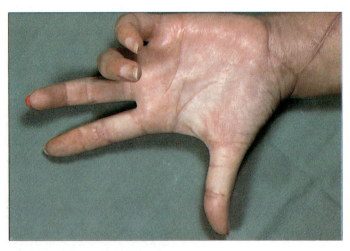

▲ 179

What lesion will cause this appearance?

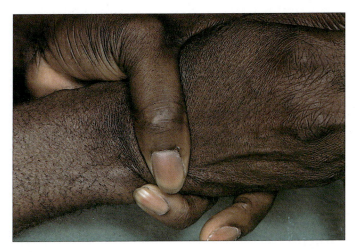

▲ 180
What diagnosis does this physical sign suggest?

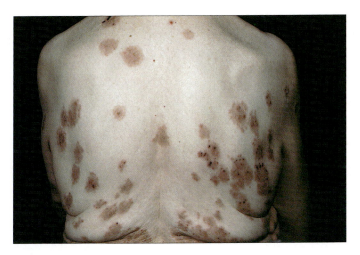

▲ 181
These papular lesions were tender and the patient had myalgia and joint effusions. What is the most likely diagnosis?

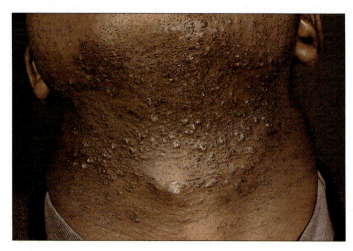

▲ 182
What is the most likely cause of this appearance?

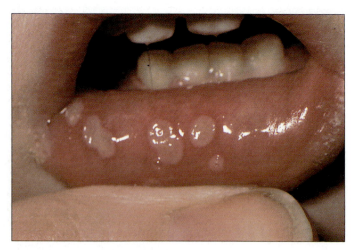

▲ 183
What is the most likely cause of these painful lesions?

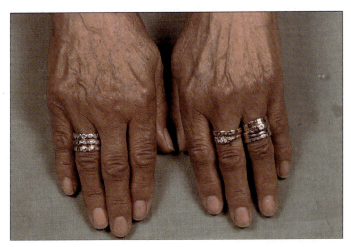

▲ **184**

This lady, with a past history of Cushing's disease, complained of progressive darkening of her skin. What is the most likely diagnosis?

**185** ▶

What are the three potential causes of this physical sign?

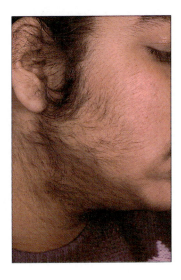

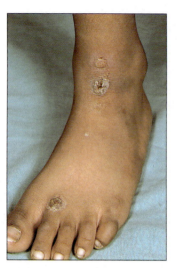

◀ **186**
What is the most likely cause of these migrating lesions?

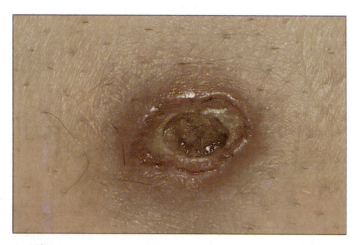

▲ **187**
This lesion appeared in a patient who had recently been on a trip to Africa. What is the most likely diagnosis?

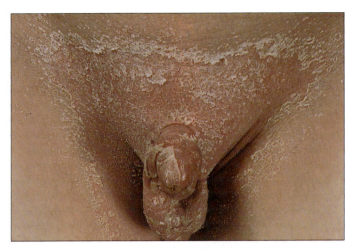

▲ 188
This patient had some oral lesions, and lymphadenopathy. What is the most likely diagnosis?

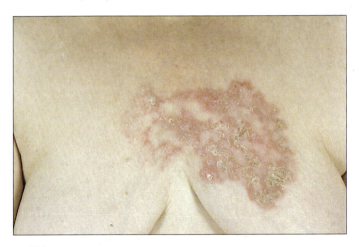

▲ 189
This lesion was insidious in onset, and first started as a deep nodule, which slowly developed into a plaque as it coalesced with neighbouring lesions. It ultimately ulcerated. What is the most likely diagnosis?

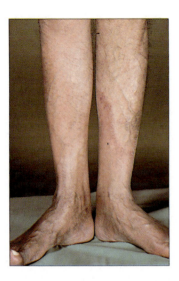

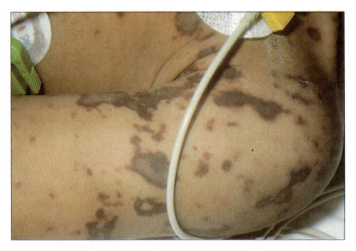

◄ 190
The lesion demonstrated was associated with a thickened peripheral nerve. What is the most likely diagnosis?

▲ 191
This patient was on a life-support machine. What is the most likely diagnosis?

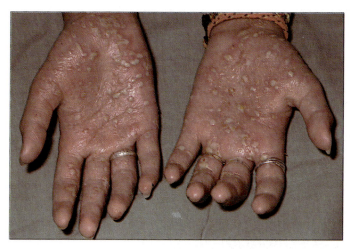

▲ 192
What physical sign is demonstrated in these hands?

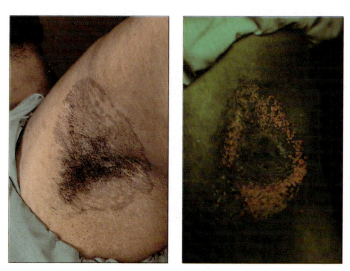

▲ 193
These two illustrations are of the same lesion, the one on the right following application of a Wood's lamp. What is the diagnosis?

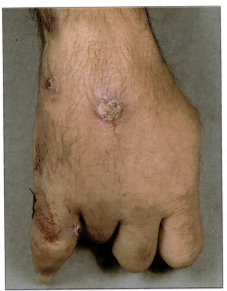

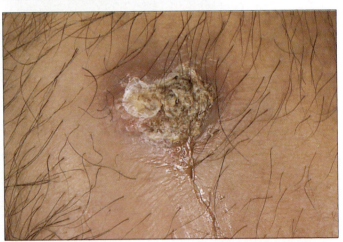

◀ ▼ 194
These two illustrations show the same chronic lesion. What is the most likely diagnosis?

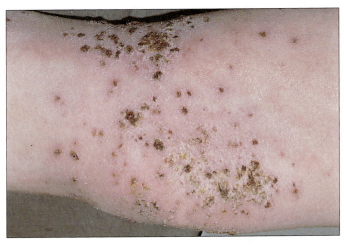

▲ 195
This patient had chronic eczema. What is the most likely cause of
this appearance?

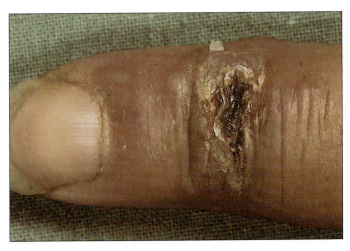

▲196
What is the most likely cause of this appearance?

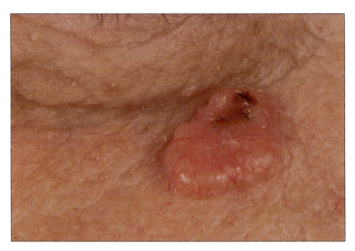

▲ **197**
What lesion is shown?

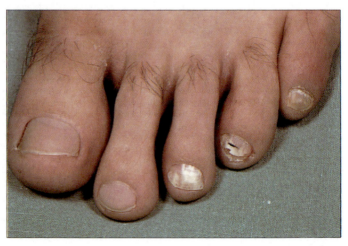

▲ **198**
What is the diagnosis?

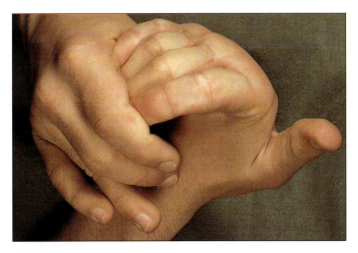

▲ 199
(a) What physical sign is shown?
(b) What are the two associations?

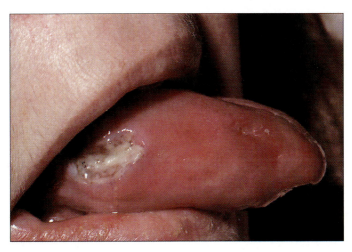

▲ 200
This is an intensely painful lesion and was associated with a sore eye. What is the most likely diagnosis?

1   Primary biliary cirrhosis.

2   (a) Acromegaly. A goitre is also present.
    (b) Patients may have carpal tunnel syndrome, as well as premature osteoarthritis.

3   Haemangioma, gynaecomastia.

4   Dissecting aortic aneurysm.

5   (a) Ophthalmic Graves' disease.
    (b) This patient has had a left tarsorrhaphy.

6   Onycholysis with Graves' disease, a fungal infection of the nails, psoriasis affecting the nails.

7   Thyroid acropachy.

8   Bowen's disease.

9   Scurvy. The features in adults include perifollicular hyperkeratotic papules in which hairs become fragmented and buried, perifollicular haemorrhages, purpura beginning on the backs of the lower extremities and coalescing to form ecchymoses, and haemorrhages into the muscles of the arms and legs with secondary phlebothromboses.

10  Rickets.

11  (a) Tendinous xanthoma.
    (b) The serum lipids should be measured.

12  Erythropoietic porphyria. The classical manifestation is cutaneous photosensitivity.

13  Xanthomata.

14  Tendinous xanthomata.

15  Xanthoma disseminatum.

16  (a) Gout.
    (b) Uric acid levels will be elevated.

17 Multiple secondary deposits in the right lung field, absent right upper limb with missing clavicle due to forelimb amputation.

18 Left hilar mass.

19 Andersen–Fabry disease.

20 Fabry's disease. This is an X-linked recessive disorder. The clinical manifestations are mainly due to intralysosomal deposits of alpha galactosyl lactosyl ceramide in the endothelial, perithelial, and smooth muscle cells of the blood vessels and in the histiocytic cells of the reticuloendothelial system. The cutaneous lesions shown here are angiokeratoma corporis diffusum. These lesions appear in childhood or around puberty and with time increase in number.

21 Sclerotic deposits in the lower lumbar spine and pelvis from prostatic carcinoma.

22 This shows a hilar mass.

23 Multiple lipomas. These could also be neurofibromas.

24 Xanthomata. The lipid levels should be checked.

25 Gouty tophi.

26 Cryoglobulinaemia. This presents as a typical hypersensitivity vasculitis confined to the skin. It may be associated with glomerulonephritis, arthralgias, hepatosplenomegaly, and lymphadenopathy, in addition to skin involvement. The cryoglobulins usually consist of a cryoprecipitable immunoglobulin (Ig) M rheumatoid factor directed against normal endogenous IgG.

27 Pseudohypoparathyroidism. Typically, there is metacarpal shortening of the fourth and fifth metacarpals.

28 Charcot's joints.

29 Rickets.

30 Paget's disease; in this instance affecting the left scapula.

31 Multiple bony deposits from prostatic carcinoma.

32 Early rheumatoid arthritis. There is periarticular osteoporosis with mild ulnar deviation and some erosive changes.

33 (a) Herpes genitalis.
(b) The patient could be treated with a course of acyclovir to reduce the duration of the clinical syndrome.

34 Cavernous haemangioma.

35 Phaeochromocytoma.

36 A blue naevus.

37 Cavernous haemangioma.

38 Thyrotoxicosis; in this case due to Graves' disease.

39 A foreign body should be excluded. In this case, a glass foreign body was buried in his foot and led to rapid infective changes and ultimately gangrene of his second toe.

40 (a) This patient has a classical myxoedematous facies.
(b) Neurological complications include carpal tunnel syndrome, drop attacks, ataxia, and neuropsychiatric complications.

41 Necrobiosis lipoidica diabeticorum.

42 Neuropathic diabetic ulcer involving the heel.

43 Suppressed. This is a Conn's adenoma.

44 Diabetic cheiroarthropathy.

45 Diabetic dermopathy.

46 Addison's disease. There is buccal pigmentation, and abnormal liver function tests are not infrequent in Addison's disease. Weight loss is almost invariable.

47 Acromegaly. There is prognathism and separation of the teeth. Another oral feature of acromegaly includes the tendency to snore due to soft tissue enlargement in the soft palate. Macroglossia may also be present.

**48** The most likely cause is testicular feminization. Although this patient has good breast growth, she has no pubic hair and her karyotype is likely to be XY.

**49** Addison's disease. He has pigmentation around his teeth. This is an infrequent site of pigmentation in Addison's disease, which more usually occurs opposite the molar teeth.

**50** (a) Striae.
(b) These are most commonly seen in Cushing's syndrome from any cause, but occasionally occur in pregnancy or during phases of very rapid growth. Under those circumstances, they are most likely to occur in the flanks rather than in the periumbilical region demonstrated here.

**51** Left upper lobe collapse. There is some compensatory emphysema and the trachea is deviated to the left.

**52** Gross lymphoedema of the lower limbs.

**53** Bronchiectasis of the left lower zone.

**54** Pellagra.

**55** Xanthomata on the hands. The lipids should be measured.

**56** Pituitary microadenoma. This coronal magnetic resonance imaging (MRI) scan shows the optic chiasm and a fairly central stalk, but with a right-sided lesion.

**57** Meningococcal meningitis.

**58** Thalassaemia major. There is extensive gum hypertrophy due to extramedullary haemopoiesis.

**59** Carotenaemia, due to an excessive intake of carrot juice.

**60** Early cytomegalovirus retinitis. This could be treated with intravenous ganciclovir.

**61** Oral candidiasis. This patient was human immunodeficiency virus (HIV)-positive.

62 Onychomycosis.

63 Intracavitary Kaposi's sarcoma.

64 (a) Trichomegaly.
   (b) This is a cutaneous manifestation of human immunodeficiency virus (HIV) disease.

65 Glossitis is shown and may be due to iron deficiency anaemia or a megaloblastic anaemia, as in this case.

66 Beta thalassaemia major, McCune–Albright syndrome. In this case, the cause was beta thalassaemia major.

67 Thrombocytopenia. In this particular case, the patient had idiopathic thrombocytopenic purpura.

68 (a) Dactylitis.
   (b) Sickle cell anaemia.

69 Haemophilia A.

70 Right fourth nerve palsy.

71 Pseudohypoparathyroidism. There is an association between hypoparathyroidism and some somatic abnormalities. These include short stature, a round face, short neck, and shortening of the metacarpals and metatarsals.

72 There has been a bleed leading to haematoma formation in the left calf. This occurred in a haemophiliac.

73 Allergic vasculitis.

74 Planar xanthomata. This suggests underlying dyslipidaemia.

75 Henoch–Schönlein (anaphylactoid) purpura.

76 A Charcot's neuropathic joint.

**77** Langerhans' cell histiocytosis. A typical histological appearance of these lesions would be consistent with the presence of histiocytes and small round cells in various proportions, together with differing numbers of eosinophils. Electron microscopy can be extremely helpful in identifying the cells as Langerhans' cells by revealing characteristic inclusion granules (Birbeck granules) in the histiocytes. The enzymes alpha mannosidase, adenosine triphosphatase, and acid phosphatase are positive in Langerhans' cells and can be helpful in diagnosis.

**78** Acromegaly. The coarsened features, prominent nasolabial fold, and enlarged nose and lips are typical.

**79** Scurvy.

**80** Left lower lobe collapse.

**81** Pterygium.

**82** Melanosis oculi.

**83** Herpes zoster involving the left eyelid. Treatment should be commenced with intravenous acyclovir.

**84** This shows a florid papilloedema.

**85** Duane syndrome. In this disorder, fibrosis of the lateral rectus muscle causes failure of abduction and retraction of the eye and ptosis on abduction. It may be unilateral or bilateral and is sometimes inherited as a dominant trait. It is occasionally associated with pseudopapilloedema and the Klippel–Feil syndrome.

**86** Polychondritis.

**87** Infective endocarditis. This shows an Osler's node.

**88** (a) Gum hypertrophy–hyperplasia.
(b) This may be associated with use of phenytoin or cyclosporin.

**89** Subacute bacterial endocarditis. There are multiple cutaneous lesions in the toes.

90 Raynaud's phenomenon.

91 Raynaud's disease.

92 Wegener's granulomatosis with a saddle nose deformity.

93 (a) Acanthosis nigricans.
(b) This may occur in acromegaly or in other insulin-resistant states, such as Roth's syndrome.

94 (a) Oral telangiectasia.
(b) Internal lesions occasionally bleed, causing iron deficiency anaemia.

95 The appearances are those of bilateral ulnar nerve lesions. There will be associated loss of sensation on the ulnar border of the hand.

96 Black hairy tongue. This occasionally occurs with tetracycline intake.

97 Crohn's disease.

98 (a) Palmar erythema.
(b) This may occur with chronic liver disease, thyrotoxicosis, and rheumatoid arthritis.

99 Cirrhosis with portal hypertension and porto-systemic shunt.

100 (a) Leuconychia.
(b) This may be associated with both liver and renal failure.

101 Nephrotic syndrome. There is bilateral pitting oedema of the lower limbs and the hypoalbuminaemia of the nephrotic syndrome is often associated with quite severe dyslipidaemia.

102 Small muscle wasting and diffuse pigmentation of the skin. This patient had chronic renal failure.

103 Dystrophia myotonica. There is quite severe wasting of the sterno-cleidomastoid muscle.

104 (a) There is ectopic calcification in the eye.
(b) This may be associated with primary hyperparathyroidism or chronic renal failure.

**105** Deviation of the tongue due to left twelfth nerve damage (lower motor neurone). When the patient pokes his tongue out, it deviates towards the weaker (affected) side if there is a unilateral upper or lower motor neurone lesion. Unilateral lower motor neurone lesions with a central cause include vascular lesions, such as thrombosis of the vertebral artery, motor neurone disease, and syringobulbia Causes in the posterior fossa include tumours, aneurysms, chronic meningitis, and trauma, and in the upper neck, syringomyelia, tumours, and the Arnold–Chiari malformation.

**106** (a) Wasting of the small muscles of the hand.
(b) This is likely to be a T1 lesion; in this case, a thoracic outlet syndrome.

**107** (a) Bilateral carpal tunnel syndrome with bilateral wasting of the abductor policis brevis.
(b) Potential causes include hypothyroidism, acromegaly, rheumatoid arthritis, as well as anterior dislocation of the lunate.

**108** (a) Clubbing and nailfold vasculitis.
(b) Subacute bacterial endocarditis.

**109** Mononeuritis affecting the ulnar nerve.

**110** S1.

**111** Charcot–Marie–Tooth disease.

**112** (a) Winged scapula.
(b) This is generally caused by weakness of the serratus anterior muscle.

**113** Diabetes mellitus and primary gonadal failure. The appearances are those of dystrophia myotonica with frontal balding, bilateral ptosis, and myopathic facies.

**114** Central retinal venous occlusion.

**115** Central retinal artery occlusion.

**116** (a) Retinitis pigmentosa.
(b) This may be associated with Batten's disease and with phenothiazine intake.

**117** A simple macular pigmentation.

118 Opaque myelinated optic nerve fibres. This is an entirely innocuous appearance.

119 (a) Retinochoroiditis.
(b) This is associated with *Toxocara* or *Toxoplasma* infection and sarcoidosis.

120 Central choroidal atrophy.

121 Simple choroidal naevus.

122 Anterior uveitis. Keratic precipitates are well shown.

123 Acute glaucoma. There is corneal oedema and a conjunctival injection.

124 Glaucoma. There is a deepened optic cup.

125 There is a retinal haemorrhage near the optic nerve.

126 Left medial rectus weakness.

127 Corneal abscess.

128 (a) Keratoconus.
(b) This may be associated with type 6 Ehlers–Danlos syndrome. There is a cone-shaped deformity of the cornea.

129 (a) Rosacea. This is a chronic inflammatory disorder involving the central area of the face and is usually seen with acneiform lesions and telangiectasias.
(b) Predisposing factors include occupational factors such as exposure to excessive sunlight or severe winds (e.g. in farmers and sailors), food (chronic alcoholism and a spicy diet may aggravate rosacea), and psychological factors (patients are usually slightly depressed, but the depression is probably due to their facial disfigurement).

130 Impetigo.

131 Impetigo.

132 Pilonidal sinus. The patient was a hairdresser.

133 (a) Pyoderma gangrenosum.
(b) This may be associated with ulcerative colitis or Crohn's disease.

134 Pyogenic granuloma. This lesion requires curetting.

135 Seborrhoeic dermatitis.

136 Pityriasis rosea. This is a mild inflammatory disease characterized by macules and maculopapular lesions, which are slightly scaly and form mostly on the trunk. The onset is sudden and heralded by the appearance of a solitary macular lesion. This is known as the herald patch and there is an interval of 7–10 days while the herald patch persists alone before other lesions appear.

137 Nodular prurigo. The nodules are 1–2 cm in diameter and scattered over extensor areas. It is sometimes a consequence of a partially resolved, more generalized pruritus due to atopic eczema or parasite infestation. Deep pigmentation may result in pigmented races.

138 Oral lichen planus. Mucous membranes are affected in 25–70% of all cases. The lesions on the inner sides of the cheek are tiny milky-white papules or are arranged in a network pattern of thin thread-like streaks. The lips, tongue, and palate may be similarly affected.

139 Lichen planus. The nails are affected in about 10% of cases, and in some patients the nails may be affected in the absence of skin lesions. The nail changes are non-specific and may appear as longitudinal furrows, which vary in depth. Ridges may be continuous with the cuticle.

140 Chronic discoid lupus erythematosus.

141 Lichen planus. The photograph demonstrates an example of Koebner's phenomenon.

142 Pityriasis alba.

143 Pityriasis rosea. This should be compared to the appearance of 136, which shows a close-up view of one of the lesions.

144 Psoriasis. The extensor surface is typically affected.

145 Psoriasis. There is onycholysis and thimble pitting. Fungal infections and Plumber's nails (thyrotoxicosis) could be part of the differential diagnosis.

146 Pustular psoriasis.

147 Psoriatic arthritis. Severe deforming arthritis sometimes occurs in psoriasis, showing widespread ankylosis or having the clinical appearance of an arthritis mutilans.

148 This is an epidermolytic staphylococcal infection (Ritter's disease).

149 Discoid lupus erythematosus.

150 Sarcoidosis (lupus pernio).

151 Lichen planus.

152 Macular amyloid.

153 Rhinophyma. Long-standing rosacea may lead to connective tissue overgrowth, particularly of the nose (rhinophyma), and may be complicated by inflammatory disorders of the eye, including keratitis, blepharitis, iritis, and recurrent chalazion.

154 Erythema nodosum.

155 This is most likely a drug-induced erythema multiforme.

156 Pemphigus.

157 Toxic epidermal necrolysis.

158 Erythema multiforme.

159 Erythema annulare.

160 Bullous pemphigoid. The bullae are subepidermal and acantholysis is not a feature. About 80% of patients are over 60 years of age and it is about twice as common as pemphigus. There is a specific antibody, usually immunoglobulin G, for the basement membrane zone of the epidermis in about 70% of patients.

161 Pemphigus vulgaris.

162 Eczema en craquelé.

163 Dermatitis herpetiformis. The lesions may also be found at the elbows and in front of the knees.

**164** Phytophotodermatitis.

**165** Fixed drug eruption.

**166** Contact dermatitis.

**167** Lip smack dermatitis.

**168** Recurrent erythema multiforme.

**169** Dermatitis herpetiformis.

**170** Disseminated intravascular coagulation, in this particular case caused by meningococcal septicaemia.

**171** Kaposi's sarcoma.

**172** Pseudopelade of Brocq.

**173** Alopecia totalis.

**174** Yellow nail syndrome.

**175** Scleral melanoma.

**176** Vitiligo. This is a non-organ-specific manifestation of autoimmune disease.

**177** Bazin's disease. This disease is characterized by symmetrical indurated nodules on the back of the legs and occasionally elsewhere. It predominates in females, usually 10–20 years of age. The pathology shows a non-specific or tuberculoid infiltrate in the lower part of the dermis. Proliferative changes occur, and caseation, which accounts for the clinical breakdown of the lesions, is also a feature.

**178** Behçet's disease.

**179** Ulnar nerve lesion.

**180** Marfan's syndrome.

**181** Sweet's syndrome: the rash is characteristic and composed of tender red or purple discrete skin plaques. The manifestations usually resolve over a 2–3-month period.

182 Pseudofolliculitis.

183 Painful aphthous ulceration. In this case the appearances were due to herpetic dermatitis.

184 Nelson's syndrome.

185 This patient has severe hirsuties, which may be caused by a virilizing tumour of the adrenal or ovary, or (as in this case) simple polycystic ovary syndrome.

186 Sporotrichosis.

187 Cutaneous leishmaniasis.

188 Kawasaki disease. The principal features are a fever lasting for five days or more, bilateral congestion of ocular conjunctivae, changes of the lips and oral cavity with fissuring and dryness of the mucous membranes, acute non-tender swelling of the cervical lymph nodes, a polymorphous exanthema, and changes of the extremities, with reddening of the palms and soles and desquamation, as in this picture.

189 Lupus vulgaris. In this lesion, the tubercle bacillus is inoculated directly into the skin. It is commoner in women than men. With diascopy, the lesion becomes white, and the nodules appear brown, having jelly-like spots in the centre.

190 Tuberculoid leprosy. The typical lesion is a plaque, which is erythematous and usually single, with a raised and well-defined edge from which there is a gradual slope towards a flattened and hypopigmented centre. The surface is dry, hairless, insensitive, and sometimes scaly, and a thickened peripheral nerve is usually palpable in the vicinity. Damage to a peripheral nerve causing a sensory or motor disturbance may precede the skin lesion.

191 Meningococcal meningitis with evidence of disseminated intravascular coagulation.

192 Infected eczema.

193 Erythrasma. This is due to a corynebacterial infection of the axillae. On white skin it is light brown, but on dark skin it may produce a lighter or darker hue. Wood's light shows the coral or red fluorescence.

**194** Actinomycosis. This is caused by an aerobic or microaerophilic *Actinomyces*. In tissues, compact mycelial growth results in the formation of characteristic colonies of ray fungus. These may be extruded from the sinuses as pale-buff sulphur granules. The apparent exudate should be carefully examined for sulphur granules, which are identified by Gram's stain.

**195** Kaposi's varicelliform eruption.

**196** Herpetic whitlow.

**197** Basal cell carcinoma. The typical rolled edges with a crusted lesion on top are characteristic.

**198** Tinea unguium.

**199** (a) Joint hyperlaxity.
(b) This may occur in Marfan's syndrome and Ehlers–Danlos syndrome.

**200** Behçet's disease.

# INDEX

Numbers refer to Question and Answer numbers.